EAT YOURSELF THIN

HEALTHY EATING FOR A SLIMMER, FITTER YOU

GODBLESS BAKPA AMREVWODJE

Copyright © 2023 GODBLESS BAKPA AMREVWODJE.

Eat Yourself Thin, Healthy Eating for a Slimmer; Fitter You is a nonfictional work. The author either created the names, characters, settings, and happenings in their own minds or utilized them in a creative manner. Any likeness to genuine individuals, living or dead, events, or locations is purely coincidental.

Table of Contents

INTRODUCTION

The breakthrough weight loss method Eating Yourself Thin emphasizes making minor adjustments to your food and way of life to help you lose weight. This strategy places a strong emphasis on mindful eating, portion control, and paying attention to the quality of the food you consume. Making tiny changes that have a large impact on your general health is what Eating Yourself Thin encourages you to do rather than excessive dieting or tight meal planning.

A comprehensive approach to weight loss called Eating Yourself Thin considers the entire individual rather than just the number on the scale.

 Finding the root causes of your weight gain is helpful, and after that, it motivates you to adjust your food and lifestyle in order to achieve your objectives. Eating Yourself Thin emphasizes making manageable, small changes that can result in long-term weight loss while also enhancing general health.

In Eating Yourself Thin, the first step is to identify the items you are currently eating and determine whether they are causing you to gain weight. You can determine which meals to eat in moderation and which to avoid with the aid of this assessment. You can concentrate on making simple dietary modifications, such as reducing portion sizes, staying away from processed meals, and favoring whole, unprocessed foods, once you've identified the foods that are causing you to gain weight.

The focus of Eating Yourself Thin's next stage will be mindful eating. Eating yourself thin encourages you to be conscious of your meal selections, to taste the flavors of your food, and to be aware of your body's hunger and fullness cues rather than mindlessly eating. Practicing mindful eating can help you avoid overeating and make sure you are getting the proper amount of nutrition for your needs.

Focusing on making tiny, doable lifestyle adjustments is the last phase in Eating Yourself Thin. This includes adopting good habits like meal planning and grocery shopping as well as engaging in regular physical activity, getting enough sleep, regulating your stress levels, and managing your time. In contrast to excessive dieting, eating oneself thin emphasizes incremental improvements that can result in long-term weight loss and improved general health.

Making manageable, small dietary and lifestyle adjustments is the main goal of the successful weight loss program Eating Yourself Thin. With an emphasis on the type of food you eat, this strategy promotes mindful eating and portion control. You can accomplish long-term weight loss and increased general health by making tiny modifications to your diet and way of life.

CHAPTER 1

The Basics of Eating Yourself Thin

In recent years, the idea of "eating yourself slim" has become more widespread. Its foundation is the notion that achieving and maintaining a healthy weight may be accomplished with the use of nutrition. Additionally, it helps you stay healthy, increase your immune system's strength, and increase your energy levels.

Making good meal choices is the main component of eating yourself thin. Selecting foods that are high in nutrients and low in calories is necessary to achieve this. Consuming a lot of lean meats, fresh produce, low-fat dairy products, and nutritious grains are all part of this. As a result of the high fiber, vitamin, and mineral content of these foods, you'll feel fuller for longer and be able to maintain a healthy weight. It may be possible to lessen bloating and water retention by eating more fiber-rich meals to maintain a healthy digestive tract.

As processed meals are frequently high in extra carbohydrates, bad fats, sodium, and calories, it's crucial to keep this in mind. Moreover, since trans and saturated fats are linked to an increased risk of heart disease, it's a good idea to limit your intake of these foods.

When eating oneself thin, you must be mindful of your portion choices in addition to choosing healthy foods. The tendency to overeat is all too common. Research has shown that people who consume fewer quantities typically lose weight more quickly and keep it off longer.

Finally, eating yourself skinny requires paying attention to what you're putting in your mouth. Knowing how certain foods make you feel and how they impact your body is necessary for this. For instance, it's preferable to stay away from a food if you know that consuming it makes you feel bloated or lethargic. Listening to your body's signals of hunger and fullness is also crucial. In order to avoid overeating, it's important to eat only when you're actually hungry and stop eating when you're full.

A healthy weight can be maintained and your general health can be enhanced by eating oneself slim. You can make good changes to your diet that will aid in achieving your weight loss objectives by selecting nutrient-dense meals, avoiding processed foods, monitoring your portion sizes, and eating mindful

CHAPTER 2

The best and most efficient way to reduce weight (permanently) and stay healthy is through proper eating. Unfortunately, the majority of weight-loss programs don't take your health into account. Let's look at some of the most common weight loss techniques that can be harmful.

1. Dietary supplements. Some are used to suppress hunger. Due to the issue not being addressed, these are ineffective for the majority of people. Even if you have a large appetite, that is not the issue. You lose water weight when taking other diet medicines. As the scales tell you a narrative, you may feel as though you are losing weight as a result. However, this might be harmful. Many people already have some level of dehydration. Again, you need to shed fat tissue, not water.

2. Calorie counting can get you into trouble. It's not just difficult; it can also influence your dietary choices. Keeping your calorie consumption under control has nothing to do with your health. You can become always hungry as a result. You won't be able to maintain a healthy diet if you don't try. Also, the weight will come back.

3. Diets high in protein are currently popular. They can assist you in losing weight, but once more at the expense of your health. Even though a diet heavy in protein can aid in weight loss in the short term, it is bad for your health in the long run. They may also restrict your consumption of nutritious foods. Does that make sense at all?

4. Diet plans that include meals always serve you in tiny portions. Your body's nutritional needs aren't met by little servings, which makes you hungry and likely to skip meals. It's not difficult to spot a significant nutritional quality fault when you look at some of the most popular dishes.

5. Bariatric surgery is the surgical implantation of a band around your stomach to physically reduce how much you can consume. These can be harmful in addition to being extremely expensive (fortunately out of the price range of many overweight people). They are subject to all the risks associated with surgery and may leave a postoperative trail of deteriorating health or even death. Gallstones or a hiatus hernia, as well as gastro-intestinal issues like indigestion, distention, nausea, and bowel dysfunction, are some of the problems. You can develop anemia and have swallowing issues. It is typical to experience severe nutritional deficiencies, which might deteriorate health.

You can expect to lose weight and experience improved health when you learn about healthy foods and which foods are unhealthy and should be avoided or at least limited.

Obesity or being overweight is a byproduct of civilization. It doesn't happen in the wild. Nutritional inadequacy is the cause of it. You might have a voracious appetite as a result of this. Learn how a permanent solution to two issues can be obtained through healthy eating for weight loss.

Five Ways for a Healthier Diet and Quicker Weight Loss

If you want to lose weight permanently, you need to have three things. They are: a healthy diet, frequent exercise, and the appropriate frame of mind. Your diet and eating habits have a significant impact on how much weight you acquire or lose. I outline five practices in this book that promote healthy eating for weight loss. Make each of these a daily habit by doing so slowly but gradually. You will have adopted a much healthier eating lifestyle before you know it. The appropriate habits must be established in order to engage in healthy eating for weight loss.

1. Breakfast is the most crucial meal of the day.

This is true, and you've undoubtedly heard it before. Your body requires nourishment to power you through the day after around ten hours of fasting. You can give your body the energy it needs for the remainder of the day by eating breakfast. After having breakfast, you'll feel more energized and aware.

2. Avoid skipping lunch

It makes sense theoretically that skipping lunch will help you lose weight more quickly. Wrong. When you skip lunch, your blood sugar levels drop, your metabolism slows to make up for the lost energy, and by the time you arrive home, you are ravenous and will eat anything that is in your path. That is the ideal recipe for gaining weight.

Never skipping lunch, or any other meal, is one of the rules of healthy eating for weight loss.

Eat modest, frequent meals throughout the day. In this manner, you avoid overeating and prevent your body from running out of energy. Savvy?

3. Frequently Snack

Never let yourself go hungry at any time, as a general rule. You must always have something in your stomach. You must provide your body the energy it requires in order for it to burn fat more effectively. You can't eat complete meals frequently, yes. Snack, but avoid junk food. You can eat fruit, nuts, pretzels, apples, and oranges as snacks. Make sure you always have something in your stomach, and eat everything you want (in moderation). Avoid going hungry.

4. Consume Lots of Water

Water makes up 70% of your body, therefore it makes sense that it would serve as your natural source of replenishment. Your body needs to remain well hydrated in order to function at its peak. Drink eight or more glasses of water each day.

Since water has no calories, it takes more energy for your body to warm it to body temperature. Your metabolism will boost as a result, accelerating your weight loss efforts. In fact, studies have shown that even consuming several glasses of ice water throughout the day will increase your metabolism by one-third.

5. Avoid eating late

An early dinner allows your body to fully digest the meal before your seven-hour sleep period. But because of our hectic schedules, we frequently feel tempted to postpone dinner.

To succeed, keep in mind that you must include each of these suggestions into your everyday routine. Currently, it takes around twenty-one days to create a new habit. Therefore, when you fall, don't kick yourself—you may, but don't kick yourself hard—just remember that you need to get back up and keep going. You should get used to it since you will likely be doing it for the rest of your life.

Finally, eating healthy to lose weight is neither hard nor complicated. You get closer to your goal by taking each step one at a time. Happy New Year!

CHAPTER 3

Unrestricted weight loss without a rigid diet or exercise routine is now possible with the help of the book Eating Yourself Thin. It is predicated on the notion that consuming particular meals can help you cut calories and, as a result, lose weight.

Due to the fact that the foods are frequently wholesome and supply nutrients that keep your body functioning normally, many people discover this type of diet to be more enduring than conventional diet programs.

Eating Yourself Thin has several advantages over popular diets, starting with the fact that it is a far healthier way to lose weight. Your calorie intake can be decreased without having to drastically limit your food options if you concentrate on consuming wholesome, healthful foods like fruits, vegetables, lean meats, and whole grains. The ability to sample a variety of meals is another benefit of Eating Yourself Thin, which can help you stay on track with your diet and keep it interesting.

The ability to enhance general health is yet another advantage of Eating Yourself Thin. By improving your general physical and mental health, eating a balanced diet can help lower your chance of contracting specific diseases. A nutritious diet can also help you feel more energised and be more productive. Your risk of acquiring obesity, diabetes, and heart disease can be effectively decreased by following the advice in Eating Yourself Thin.

It's also a terrific approach to relieve tension to Eat Yourself Thin. Cortisol is the hormone that causes stress in the body, thus eating healthy foods can help lower your body's levels of this hormone. In addition to helping you feel better, eating a nutritious diet can also help you feel less depressed and anxious. By enhancing your sleep, Eating Yourself Thin can help you feel less stressed and have better overall health.

Lastly, Eating Yourself Thin can be a fantastic strategy to cut costs. Consuming healthier foods can help you spend less on groceries and on pricey processed foods. You'll have to spend less time preparing and cooking meals if you follow the advice in Eating Yourself Thin, which can be a terrific time-saving strategy.

As a result, Eating Thin can be a terrific approach to get healthier, lose weight, manage stress, and save money. You may adjust it to suit your particular requirements, and it is a healthy and sustainable strategy to cut calories. Your entire health can be enhanced and weight loss objectives can be successfully attained with the help of Eating Yourself Thin.

So, instead of rushing out the door in the morning, take a few minutes to prepare your body the healthy meal it so richly deserves. Your body will appreciate it.

CHAPTER 4

Are you overweight and eager to reduce your weight? That is not unusual. Are you considering starving yourself in order to lose weight? That is also not unusual. However, there are few people who are interested in losing weight without giving up foods they enjoy (such as bread, potatoes, rice, and so on).

To lose weight, you don't have to follow a strict food plan. Simply maintain a positive view on life, your weight loss plan included, and resolve to lead a better lifestyle. Make a small diet adjustment to get fit in a healthy approach. Wait! Don't stop eating, but do stop eating as much of something or as one kind of something.

To learn what you must eat and what you shouldn't in order to get back in shape, you can only consult an expert. However, following a low-calorie diet won't benefit your health in the long run. It's possible that you'll lose muscle while losing absolutely no fat. You might also omit vital nutrients, endangering your risk of under-eating and frailty. You might even gain back the weight you lost in the end. And keep in mind that diseases thrive in an unhealthy body.

What you must do to reduce weight?

Why do you give food to your body? This is done so that you will feel energized. Your body nevertheless stores the additional energy as fat. Additionally, if you binge eat, the extra fat causes you to gain weight. On the other hand, you have to burn tons of fat to lose weight.

The answer is a combination of a low-calorie diet and greater activity. According to experts, those who follow this diet successfully maintain their health.

Slowly implement changes

Less is more, so the saying goes. You must concur.

To your surprise, eating just one additional biscuit a week, for example, has the potential to cause you to gain a significant amount of weight in a year. You would be able to lose that much weight if you stopped eating the extra biscuit. The same holds true for all other items you regularly consume in excess of what is required.

It would never be effective to suddenly start exercising vigorously to lose weight. Running a few miles per day after years of inactivity is just bungling. You expose yourself to the risk of injury. Start out slowly and progressively raise the intensity of your workout.

Concentrate more on exercising than diets.

Maintain your calorie consumption, but make sure you schedule exercise. Miracles and magic really occur! You are certain to experience the most beautiful method of losing weight while enriching your entire live with consistent exercise and a healthy diet.

No requirement to use a gym. Lose weight quickly and easily! Lose weight in a better manner! Use the gentle exercise strategy! All you need to start with is a little area. A walk is also beneficial. Exercise at your leisure whatever you like—swim, run, or bike. Without a doubt, this is the natural approach to burn calories.

Purchasing this weekend? Why drive to a store in your car? You can stand on two sound legs. Does Gotta make it to your office building's fourth floor? Why utilize a lift? Employ stairs. Why watch every commercial when watching a daily soap? Rise and take a short stroll, perhaps to the kitchen for a glass of water. Do you not consider these methods to be some natural weight loss treatments?

Resilience is essential.

The outcomes will demonstrate this not right away but without a doubt. In a week or two, perhaps. Don't give up. Being patient is necessary. You must hold onto it. It's crucial to persevere. Respect it. Maintain your motivation.

Chill. Don't be afraid to try unfamiliar foods. After all, appearance is unimportant. The only thing that matters is whether or not you are healthy and capable. Create a life that is truly deserving!

CHAPTER 5

Meal Planning for Weight Loss

Day 1:

Breakfast: Oatmeal with fruit and nuts

Lunch: Salad with grilled chicken

Snack: Greek yogurt with berries

Dinner: Vegetable stir-fry with brown rice

Day 2:

Breakfast: Avocado toast with a poached egg

Lunch: Grilled salmon with quinoa and roasted vegetables.

Snack: Hummus and carrots

Dinner: Baked cod with roasted broccoli

Day 3:

Breakfast: Smoothie with banana, berries, Greek yogurt, and nuts

Lunch: Turkey wrap with lettuce, tomato, and hummus

Snack: Apple slices with nut butter

Dinner: Grilled chicken with roasted sweet potatoes and green beans

Day 4:

Breakfast: Egg scramble with tomatoes and spinach

Lunch: Quinoa bowl with grilled vegetables and feta cheese

Snack: Celery and peanut butter

Dinner: will be baked salmon over brown rice with steamed asparagus.

Day 5:

Breakfast: Overnight oats with fruit and nuts

Lunch: Lentil soup with a side salad

Snack: Kale chips

Dinner: Baked chicken with roasted cauliflower and quinoa

Day 6:

Breakfast: consists of whole-wheat bread with banana and peanut butter.

Lunch: Chickpea salad with avocado, tomato, and cucumber

Snack: Veggie sticks with hummus

Dinner: Grilled shrimp with couscous and roasted vegetables

Day 7:

Breakfast: Greek yogurt with berries and granola

Lunch: Tuna salad with crackers

Snack: Popcorn

Dinner: Vegetable stir-fry with tofu and brown rice

CHAPTER 6

A good diet must be continued if you want to lose weight permanently. Here are some pointers for creating wholesome eating practices:

1. Consume a healthy balanced diet: Include a mix of fruits, vegetables, whole grains, lean protein, and healthy fats in your diet. Steer clear of processed foods, sugary beverages, and excessive amounts of saturated and trans fats.

2. Control portion sizes: Use smaller plates and avoid overeating by eating slowly and paying attention to your body's hunger and fullness signals.

3. Avoid skipping meals: Skipping meals can lead to overeating later in the day and can slow down your metabolism.

4. Stay hydrated: Drink plenty of water throughout the day to stay hydrated and to help control hunger.

5. Plan ahead: Plan your meals and snacks in advance to ensure you have healthy options available when you're short on time.

6. Be mindful of eating out: Restaurants often serve large portions and use more oil and sugar than you would use at home. Ask for dressings and sauces on the side, and opt for grilled or baked options.

7. Get enough sleep: Lack of sleep can disrupt hormones that regulate hunger, making it harder to control cravings and overeating.

8. Exercise regularly: Regular physical activity can help boost weight loss, maintain weight loss, and improve overall health.

9. Avoid fad diets: Crash diets and other fad diets may help you lose weight quickly, but they are not sustainable and can be harmful to your health.

10. Be consistent: Weight loss and maintenance is a journey, not a destination. Be consistent with healthy eating and exercise habits to maintain your weight loss over time.

11. Keep track of your progress: Keep track of your weight and measurements, and take progress photos to help you stay motivated and on track.

12. Practice mindful eating: Pay attention to your food, chew slowly and savor each bite. By doing so, you may be able to eat less and enjoy your food more.

13. Don't eat in front of the TV or computer: Eating while you're distracted can lead to overeating and not realizing how much you've consumed.

14. Limit added sugars and saturated fats: Consuming too much added sugars and saturated fats can lead to weight gain and other health problems. Read nutrition labels and be mindful of the amount of these ingredients in the foods you eat.

15. Eat at regular intervals: Eating at regular intervals throughout the day can help prevent overeating and keep your metabolism running smoothly.

16. Find healthy replacements: Find healthy replacements for your favorite high-calorie foods to help curb cravings and make it easier to stick to your diet.

17. Get support: Reach out to friends and family for support, or consider joining a weight loss support group. Having a support system can make the weight loss journey easier.

18. Be patient: Remember that weight loss is a gradual process and it takes time to see results. Don't get discouraged if you don't see immediate changes, stay consistent and the results will come.

19. Don't restrict too much: Restricting certain foods can lead to overeating and binges. Allow yourself to have small treats in moderation, so you don't feel deprived.

20. Consult a professional: If you need help or have specific dietary needs, consider consulting a registered dietitian or nutritionist to help you create a personalized meal plan and achieve your weight loss goals.

CHAPTER 7

All weight loss programs must include exercise. It contributes to bettering overall health and wellbeing in addition to burning calories and assisting in muscle growth. The different strategies that exercise can be used to help you reach and maintain a healthy weight will be covered in this chapter.

Exercise is a fantastic means of burning calories, first and foremost. Your body uses energy to power the movement when you exercise. Your ability to burn calories increases with the intensity of your exercise. In light of this, calorie-burning exercises like jogging, cycling, and weightlifting are all fantastic choices for shedding pounds. Regular exercise can also aid to increase metabolism, which will enable you to burn calories more effectively even when you're not exercising.

Muscle development is aided by exercise. Your muscles become weakened as a result of the stress you apply to them while exercising. However, they get stronger and denser as a result of healing and reconstruction. In turn, a higher metabolism follows as muscle mass rises as a result of this. More calories are burned even when you're at rest if you have a higher metabolism. The reason why this is significant is because muscular tissue consumes more calories than fat tissue.

Additionally, physical activity can support bettering general health and wellbeing. It has been demonstrated that regular exercise reduces the risk of developing a number of diseases, including type 2 diabetes, heart disease, and stroke. Stress is lessened, mood is lifted, and energy levels are raised.

Exercise needs to become a consistent part of your routine if you want to lose weight and keep it off. On most days of the week, try to exercise for at least 30 minutes at a moderate intensity. In addition, you can divide this up into smaller, easier-to-manage time blocks, like daily ten-minutes. walks. In order to keep your workouts interesting and challenging, it's also crucial to vary them.

Finally, any regimen for losing weight must include exercise. It not only helps you lose weight but also builds muscle, enhances general health, and makes you feel better. You may achieve and maintain a healthy weight while elevating your general quality of life if you make exercise a regular part of your routine.

We all want to look our best when summer is approaching, right? so that you can visit the beach without feeling self-conscious. A lot of individuals decide to start fad diets shortly before summer arrives, but nothing changes as a result. They lose a small amount of water weight, which they quickly regain. This flat stomach diet is necessary if you want to lose weight permanently.

1. Sip a lot of water: The ideal water to drink is clean, naturally filtered water since it will assist flush out the toxins that collect around fat and keep it largely concentrated around the waist. We all understand the value of water, but do you consume the recommended eight glasses daily?

TIP: Purchase a two-liter bottle and take it to work. during the day, finish it! If you have to replenish it, you receive additional bonus points for fat loss.

2. Increase your consumption of fiber: Fiber serves a variety of purposes, including making you feel fuller and improving the efficiency of your digestive system. As a result of feeling fuller after eating less and your digestive system operating correctly, you burn fat more quickly.

TIP - Settle for a hearty bowl of fiber-rich oats instead of bread or a bowl of cornflakes. Whole meal versions of white pasta, white bread, and rice should be used instead. Aim to increase the number of pulses and legumes in your diet.

3. Take frequent, smaller, balanced meals: If you don't eat five to six meals a day, at portions that keep you full until your next meal in two to three hours, you're enabling your metabolism to slow down and your energy levels to get depleted. Switch from three square meals each day to five or six smaller meals to burn fat more quickly.

TIP - Always keep a supply of wholesome snacks on hand, and schedule when you'll need them in advance. This will reduce your need to buy quick snacks and junk food, which will not only improve your mood but also make your stomach appear flatter.

If you adhere to these flat stomach diet recommendations, getting a thin figure won't be tough. Want a flat tummy more quickly? Simply add some daily exercise to the mix. It doesn't matter what you do, as long as you move more than you would while sitting in an office.

Do you desire it? What do you see? Do you perceive it? Imagine being able to possess it. That's how easy it is. Everything begins in the mind. What a man can imagine and believe, he can accomplish.

Consider this. It all begins with a thought. "A man thinks what he becomes" What you focus on, you manifest. What you envision and consider will manifest in your life. Consider what you desire, not what you disapprove of.

Here are some suggestions to aid in maintaining a healthy weight and accomplishing your objective. Do this day and night for thirty days, and it will get ingrained in your subconscious mind, transforming you into a new person. It's crucial to repeat the advice twice daily and to do it with feeling in order for them to stick.

Use your imagination to visualize yourself at your goal weight right before you wake up in the morning and right before you go to sleep at night.

Imagine yourself at the weight you desire. Visualize your appearance in a smaller clothing. Take note of your slimmer hips and smaller waist. You become aware of your cheekbones and hip bones. While looking at your side view, you are also very pleased with your newly flat abdomen.

Observe how you feel when you are at your regular weight. Feel your energy level rise. Imagine yourself engaging in activities you've been wanting to do. Feel how effortless breathing and moving are when engaging in your favorite activities. Once you reach your healthy weight, notice how your steps become lighter and more airy. Feel how happy and pleased you feel of yourself for making the effort to appreciate and care for your body. You now want to move around more, exercise more, and select healthy foods over bad ones. When you are sufficiently nourished, you can quit eating. You only need a very small amount of bad meals to make you feel full. You are so relieved that you have control over your diet.

Pay attention to the complements that your loved ones and friends give you. You hear them expressing their pride in you for taking the necessary efforts to transform into your new, healthier you. They are telling you to keep up the good work, so hear them. Hear them compliment your appearance and inquire about your weight loss strategy. Now is the perfect time to share your weight-control advice with someone else. Hear yourself discussing the lessons you've learnt about managing your weight.

Take note of how food now tastes. Imagine yourself consuming wholesome foods like fruits, vegetables, chicken, fish, low-fat dairy, whole-wheat bread, and cereal. Take note of how much you truly like the sweet flavor, juiciness, and crunch of fresh fruits and vegetables. Now that you are eating low-fat meats and fish, take note of how much better your digestion functions. Take note of how much water you're consuming, which hydrates and cleanses your body. Healthy eating tastes fantastic and improves your appearance and well-being.

Now that you are at your target healthy weight, take note of your increased awareness. You now want to maintain your weight loss. You enjoy being active and moving about. You will never go back once you contrast how wonderful you feel right now with how you felt in the past. You now declare, "I eat to survive." 'I like my life,' I cherish being at my ideal weight. I am making an effort to stay at my optimum weight going ahead. "I am and I know I can!"

CHAPTER 8

RECIPES

BREAKFAST:

1. Overnight Oats with Fruit:

Ingredients:

Half cup rolled oats

Half cup milk (dairy or non-dairy)

Half cup diced fresh fruit of your choice

One tablespoon honey

One tablespoon chia seeds (optional)

Instructions:

1. In a bowl, combine the oats, milk, fruit, honey, and chia seeds (if using).

2. Stir until everything is thoroughly combined.

3. Place the bowl in the refrigerator overnight covered.

4. Stir the oats and enjoy them in the morning.

Prep Time: Five minutes

2. Egg White Omelet with Spinach:

Ingredients:

Four egg whites

One tablespoon olive oil

One-fourth cup diced onion

Half cup diced fresh spinach

Salt and pepper, to taste

Instructions:

1. The egg whites should be whisked together in a bowl.

2. Over medium heat, warm the olive oil in a medium skillet.

3. Cook the onion after being added until it is tender.

4. For an additional one-two minutes, add the spinach and continue to cook.

5. Pour the egg whites into the pan and cook, stirring occasionally, until the eggs are cooked through.

6. To taste, add salt and pepper to the dish.

7. Serve immediately.

Prep Time: Ten minutes

3. Breakfast Smoothie Bowl:

Ingredients:

Half cup frozen fruit of your choice

One-fourth cup plain yogurt

One-fourth cup unsweetened almond milk

One tablespoon almond butter

One teaspoon chia seeds

Instructions:

1. In a blender, combine the frozen fruit, yogurt, almond milk, almond butter, and chia seeds.

2. Blend until smooth.

3. Pour into a bowl and top with additional fruit, nuts, or seeds, if desired.

4. Enjoy immediately.

Prep Time: Five minutes

4. Banana Pancakes:

Ingredients:

One ripe banana

Two eggs

One-fourth teaspoon baking powder

Pinch of salt

Instructions:

1. Use a fork to thoroughly mash the banana in a medium bowl.

2. Add the eggs, baking powder, and salt and whisk until combined.

3. Heat a non-stick skillet over medium heat and lightly grease with butter or oil.

4. Pour the batter into the pan and cook for one-two minutes, or until the bottom is lightly golden.

5. Cook for an additional one-two minutes after flipping.

6. Serve with your favorite toppings.

Prep Time: Ten minutes

5. Avocado Toast:

Ingredients:

Two slices whole wheat bread

Half avocado, mashed

One-fourth teaspoon garlic powder

Salt and pepper, to taste

Instructions:

1. Toast the bread until lightly golden.

2. Use a fork to mash the avocado in a small bowl..

3. Stir in the garlic powder and season with salt and pepper, to taste.

4. Spread the avocado over the toast and enjoy.

Prep Time: Five minutes

6. Baked Egg Cups:

Ingredients:

Six eggs

One-fourth cup diced bell pepper

One-fourth cup diced onion

One-fourth cup diced ham

Salt and pepper, to taste

Instructions:

1. Preheat the oven to 375°F.

2. Grease a muffin pan just a little with butter or oil.

3. The eggs should be beaten together in a medium bowl.

4. Add the ham, onion, and bell pepper.

5. To taste, add salt and pepper to the dish.

6. Evenly distribute the mixture among the muffin tin cups.

7. Bake the egg cups for fifteen-twenty minutes, or until they are set..

8. Serve warm.

Prep Time: Ten minutes

7. Greek Yogurt Parfait:

Ingredients:

Half cup plain Greek yogurt

One-fourth cup granola

One-fourth cup diced fresh fruit of your choice

Instructions:

1. In a bowl, layer the yogurt, granola, and fruit.

2. Repeat with additional layers until the bowl is full.

3. Enjoy immediately.

Prep Time: Five minutes

8. Avocado Egg Boats:

Ingredients:

Two avocados

Four eggs

One-fourth cup diced tomatoes

One-fourth cup shredded cheese

Salt and pepper, to taste

Instructions:

1. Preheat the oven to 375°F.

2. Remove the pits from the avocados before cutting them in half.

3. The avocados should be placed on a baking dish.

4. Each half of an avocado should contain an egg.

5. Top with the tomatoes and cheese.

6. To taste, add salt and pepper to the dish.

7. Bake for about fifteen and twenty minutes, or until the eggs are fully cooked..

8. Serve warm.

Prep Time: Ten minutes

9. Breakfast Burrito:

Ingredients:

One-fourth cup cooked black beans

One-fourth cup diced bell pepper

One-fourth cup diced onion

Two eggs

Two tablespoons shredded cheese

One small whole wheat tortilla

Instructions:

1. In a medium skillet, heat the black beans, bell pepper, and onion over medium heat.

2. Cook until the vegetables are softened.

3. Add the eggs and stir until they are fully cooked..

4. Remove the mixture from the heat and stir in the cheese.

5. Place the mixture onto the tortilla and roll up.

Enjoy immediately.

Prep Time: Ten minutes

10. Breakfast Tacos:

Ingredients:

One-fourth cup cooked black beans

One-fourth cup diced bell pepper

One-fourth cup diced onion

Two eggs

Two tablespoons shredded cheese

Two small corn tortillas

Instructions:

1. In a medium skillet, heat the black beans, bell pepper, and onion over medium heat.

2. Cook until the vegetables are softened.

3. Add the eggs and scramble them until fully cooked.

4. Remove the mixture from the heat and stir in the cheese.

5. Divide the mixture between the two tortillas and top with additional toppings, if desired.

Enjoy immediately.

Prep Time: Ten minutes

LUNCH

1. Grilled Salmon with Spinach and Feta:

Ingredients:

Four ounces skinless salmon fillets,

Two tablespoons olive oil

Salt and pepper, to taste

One cup fresh spinach

Two tablespoons crumbled feta cheese

Instructions:

1. Preheat grill to medium-high heat.

2. Apply oil to the salmon and sprinkle salt and pepper over it.

3. Grill salmon for four to six minutes per side, or until cooked through.

4. Meanwhile, in a medium bowl, combine spinach and feta cheese.

5. Serve salmon with spinach and feta mixture.

Prep Time: Ten minutes

2. Chicken, Broccoli, and Brown Rice Bowl:

Ingredients:

Two cups cooked brown rice

Two tablespoons olive oil

Cut into cubes, one pound of boneless, skinless chicken breasts

Two cloves garlic, minced

One teaspoon dried oregano

Half teaspoon paprika

One-fourth teaspoon salt

Two cups broccoli florets

Instructions:

1. Over medium-high heat, warm the oil in a large skillet.

2. Add chicken, garlic, oregano, paprika, and salt. Cook, stirring occasionally, until chicken is cooked through, about five minutes.

3. Add broccoli and cook until tender, about three minutes.

4. Divide cooked rice and chicken-broccoli mixture into four bowls and serve.

Prep Time: fifteen minutes

3. Greek Quinoa Salad:

Ingredients:

One cup quinoa, cooked

Half cup cherry tomatoes, halved

Half cup cucumber, diced

One-fourth cup red onion, diced

One-fourth cup kalamata olives, sliced

Two tablespoons fresh parsley, chopped

Two tablespoons olive oil

Two tablespoons lemon juice

Instructions:

1. In a large bowl, combine quinoa, tomatoes, cucumber, red onion, olives, and parsley.

2. Mix the lemon juice and olive oil in a small bowl.

3. Pour dressing over quinoa mixture and toss to combine.

4. Serve chilled or at room temperature.

Prep Time: Ten minutes

4. Avocado and Egg Toast:

Ingredients:

Two slices whole wheat bread, toasted

Half avocado, mashed

Two eggs, cooked to your liking

Salt and pepper, to taste

Instructions:

1. Spread mashed avocado onto toast.

2. Top each slice of toast with an egg.

3. Pepper and salt should be added to taste.

Prep Time: Ten minutes

5. Zucchini Noodle Bowl with Grilled Chicken:

Ingredients:

Two cups spiralized zucchini noodles

One tablespoon olive oil

Half pound boneless skinless chicken breasts

Salt and pepper, to taste

Half cup cherry tomatoes, halved

Two tablespoons crumbled feta cheese

Instructions:

1. Preheat grill to medium-high heat.

2. Salt and pepper the chicken after brushing it with oil.

3. Grill chicken for four to six minutes per side, or until cooked through.

4. Meanwhile, in a large bowl, combine zucchini noodles, tomatoes, and feta cheese.

5. Slice chicken and add to bowl.

 Serve warm.

Prep Time: Ten minutes

6. Baked Sweet Potato Fries:

Ingredients:

 Cut into fries, two big sweet potatoes

Two tablespoons olive oil

One teaspoon smoked paprika

Half teaspoon garlic powder

Salt and pepper, to taste

Instructions:

1. Preheat oven to 425°F.

2. A baking sheet should be lined with parchment paper.

3. In a large bowl, combine sweet potato fries, olive oil, smoked paprika, garlic powder, and salt and pepper.

4. Arrange sweet potato fries on baking sheet in a single layer.

5. Bake for twenty to twenty five minutes, or until golden brown and crispy.

Prep Time: Ten minutes

7. Turkey Salad Stuffed Avocado:

Ingredients:

Two avocados, halved and pitted

Two cups cooked turkey, shredded

Two tablespoons olive oil

Two tablespoons red wine vinegar

Two tablespoons chopped fresh parsley

Salt and pepper, to taste

Instructions:

1. Scoop out the flesh of the avocados and place in a medium bowl.

2. Add turkey, olive oil, red wine vinegar, and parsley.

3. Mash with a fork until combined.

4. To taste, add salt and pepper to the meal.

5. Divide mixture among avocado halves.

Prep Time: Ten minutes

8. Kale and Quinoa Salad:

Ingredients:

One cup cooked quinoa

Two cups kale, chopped

Half cup cherry tomatoes, halved

Two tablespoons olive oil

Two tablespoons lemon juice

Salt and pepper, to taste

Instructions:

1. In a large bowl, combine quinoa, kale, and tomatoes.

2. Olive oil and lemon juice should be mixed together in a small bowl.

3. Pour dressing over quinoa mixture and toss to combine.

4. To taste, add salt and pepper to the meal.

5. Serve chilled or at room temperature.

Prep Time: Ten minutes

9. Greek Yogurt with Berries and Nuts:

Ingredients:

One cup plain Greek yogurt

Half cup fresh berries

Two tablespoons chopped nuts (almonds, walnuts, or pecans)

Two tablespoons honey

Instructions:

1. In a medium bowl, combine yogurt, berries, and nuts.

2. Drizzle with honey and stir to combine.

3. Serve chilled.

Prep Time: Five minutes

10. Shrimp and Asparagus Stir-Fry:

Ingredients:

Two tablespoons olive oil

One pound shrimp, peeled and deveined

Two cloves garlic, minced

One teaspoon fresh ginger, grated

Half teaspoon red pepper flakes

One bunch asparagus, trimmed and cut into two-inch pieces

Salt and pepper, to taste

Instructions:

1. Over medium-high heat, warm the oil in a large skillet.

2. Add shrimp and cook until just pink, about 3 minutes.

3.   Add garlic, ginger, and red pepper flakes. Cook for about a minute while stirring continuously until aromatic.

4.   Add asparagus and cook until just tender, about four minutes.

5. To taste, add salt and pepper to the meal.

6. Serve warm.

Prep Time: Ten minutes

DINNER

1. Mediterranean Baked Fish:

Ingredients:

Two (four-ounce) white fish fillets

Two tablespoons olive oil

Two cloves garlic, minced

Two tablespoons fresh lemon juice

Two tablespoons capers

Two tablespoons fresh parsley, chopped

One-fourth teaspoon salt

One-fourth teaspoon black pepper

Instructions:

1. Preheat oven to 425 degrees F.

2. Place fish fillets in a baking dish.

3. Drizzle olive oil over the fish.

4. Sprinkle garlic, lemon juice, capers, parsley, salt, and pepper over the fish.

5. Bake in preheated oven until fish flakes easily with a fork, about fifteen minutes.

Pre-time: Ten minutes

2. Chicken and Veggie Stir Fry:

Ingredients:

One tablespoon olive oil

One boneless, skinless chicken breast cut into thin strips, half cup sliced mushrooms

Half cup diced bell peppers

One-fourth cup diced onion

Two cloves garlic, minced

One teaspoon fresh ginger, minced

Two tablespoons low sodium soy sauce

Instructions:

1. Over medium-high heat, warm the oil in a large skillet.

2. Add chicken and cook until lightly browned, about five minutes.

3. Add mushrooms, bell peppers, onion, garlic, and ginger.

4. Cook until vegetables are tender-crisp, about five minutes.

5. Pour soy sauce over the stir fry.

6. Cook until chicken is cooked through and vegetables are tender, about three minutes more.

Pre-time: Ten minutes

3. Egg White Frittata:

Ingredients:

Two tablespoons olive oil

Half cup diced onion

Half cup diced bell pepper

Two cloves garlic, minced,

Six egg whites

One-fourth teaspoon salt

One-fourth teaspoon black pepper

One-fourth cup shredded cheddar cheese

Instructions:

1. Preheat oven to 350 degrees F.

2. Heat oil in a medium oven-safe skillet over medium heat.

3. Add onion, bell pepper, and garlic. Cook for about five minutes, or until vegetables are soft.

4. In a medium bowl, whisk together egg whites, salt, and pepper.

5. Over the veggies in the skillet, pour the egg mixture.

6. Cook until edges are lightly browned, about five minutes.

7. Sprinkle cheese over egg mixture.

8. Bake in preheated oven until eggs are cooked through, about fifteen minutes.

Pre-time: Ten minutes

4. Grilled Salmon with Avocado Salsa:

Ingredients:

Two (four-ounce) wild salmon fillets

 Two tablespoons olive oil

One-fourth teaspoon salt

One-fourth teaspoon black pepper

One-fourth avocado, diced

One-fourth cup diced red onion

 Two tablespoons chopped fresh cilantro

Two tablespoons fresh lime juice

Instructions:

1. Preheat a grill to medium-high heat.

2. Brush salmon fillets with olive oil and sprinkle with salt and pepper.

3. Grill salmon until cooked through, about 5 minutes per side.

4. In a medium bowl, combine avocado, red onion, cilantro, and lime juice.

5. Serve salmon with avocado salsa.

Pre-time: Ten minutes

5. Turkey and Vegetable Stir Fry:

Ingredients:

One tablespoon olive oil

One boneless, skinless turkey breast, cut into thin strips

Half cup sliced mushrooms

Half cup diced bell peppers

One-fourth cup diced onion

Two cloves garlic, minced

One teaspoon fresh ginger, minced

Two tablespoons low sodium soy sauce

Instructions:

1. In a sizable skillet, heat the oil over medium-high heat.

2. Add turkey and cook until lightly browned, about 5 minutes.

3. Add mushrooms, bell peppers, onion, garlic, and ginger.

4. Cook until vegetables are tender-crisp, about 5 minutes.

5. Pour soy sauce over the stir fry.

6. Cook until turkey is cooked through and vegetables are tender, about three minutes more.

Pre-time: Ten minutes

6. Baked Tofu with Veggies:

Ingredients:

One (fourteen-ounce) package extra-firm tofu, drained and cubed

Two tablespoons olive oil

Half cup diced bell peppers

Half cup diced onion

Two cloves garlic, minced

Two tablespoons low sodium soy sauce

Instructions:

1. Set oven to 375 degrees Fahrenheit.

2. Place tofu cubes in a baking dish.

3. Drizzle olive oil over the tofu.

4. Sprinkle bell peppers, onion, garlic, and soy sauce over the tofu.

5. Bake in preheated oven until tofu is lightly browned and vegetables are tender, about twenty minutes.

Pre-time: Ten minutes

7. Grilled Chicken with Spinach Salad:

Ingredients:

Two tablespoons olive oil

Two boneless, skinless chicken breasts

One-fourth teaspoon salt

One-fourth teaspoon black pepper

Two cups spinach

One-fourth cup diced red onion

Two tablespoons apple cider vinegar

One tablespoon honey

Instructions:

1. Preheat a grill to medium-high heat.

2. Olive oil should be used to coat the chicken before adding salt and pepper.

3. Grill chicken until cooked through, about five minutes per side.

4. In a large bowl, combine spinach, red onion, vinegar, and honey.

5. Toss to combine. Serve chicken with spinach salad.

Pre-time: Ten minutes

8. Turkey and Spinach Stuffed Peppers:

Ingredients:

Two bell peppers, halved and seeded

One tablespoon olive oil

Half cup diced onion

Half cup diced mushrooms

Two cloves garlic, minced

Half pound ground turkey

One-fourth teaspoon salt

One-fourth teaspoon black pepper

Two cups spinach

Instructions:

1. Preheat oven to 350 degrees F.

2. Place pepper halves in a baking dish.

3. Over medium heat, warm the oil in a big skillet.

4. Add onion and mushrooms and cook until vegetables are tender, about five minutes.

5. Add garlic and turkey and cook until turkey is cooked through, about five minutes more.

6. Add salt, pepper, and spinach and cook until spinach is wilted, about two minutes more.

7. Spoon mixture into pepper halves.

8. Bake in preheated oven until peppers are tender, about twenty five minutes.

Pre-time: Ten minutes

9. Shrimp and Rice Bowl:

Ingredients:

Two tablespoons olive oil

Half pound shrimp, peeled and deveined

One-fourth teaspoon salt

One-fourth teaspoon black pepper

Half cup uncooked white rice

One cup low-sodium vegetable broth

Half cup diced bell pepper

Half cup diced onion

Instructions:

1. On medium heat, warm the oil in a big skillet.

2. Add shrimp, salt, and pepper.

3. Cook until shrimp are pink and cooked through, about 5 minutes.

4. Add rice, broth, bell pepper, and onion.

5. Bring to a boil, reduce heat to low, cover, and simmer until rice is cooked through, about fifteen minutes.

Pre-time: Ten minutes

10. Grilled Vegetable Skewers:

Ingredients:

Two tablespoons olive oil

Half cup diced bell peppers

Half cup diced mushrooms

Half cup diced onion

Half teaspoon salt

Half teaspoon black pepper

Instructions:

1. Preheat a grill to medium-high heat.

2. Thread bell peppers, mushrooms, and onion onto skewers.

3. Apply olive oil to the surface and season with salt and pepper.

 4. Grill until vegetables are tender, about 5 minutes per side.

Pre-time: Ten minutes

11. Tomato and Basil Bruschetta:

Ingredients:

One French baguette, cut into twelve slices

Two tablespoons olive oil

Two cloves garlic, minced

Four tomatoes, diced

One-fourth cup fresh basil, chopped

One-fourth teaspoon salt

One-fourth teaspoon black pepper

Instructions:

1. Preheat oven to 350 degrees F.

2. On a baking sheet, arrange the baguette slices.

3. Brush with olive oil and sprinkle with garlic.

4. Bake in preheated oven until lightly browned, about ten minutes.

5. In a medium bowl, combine tomatoes, basil, salt, and pepper.

6. Top each baguette slice with tomato mixture.

Pre-time: Ten minutes

12. Grilled Salmon with Mango Salsa:

Ingredients:

Two (four-ounce) wild salmon fillets

Two tablespoons olive oil

One-fourth teaspoon salt

One-fourth teaspoon black pepper

One mango, diced

One-fourth cup diced red onion

Two tablespoons chopped fresh cilantro

Two tablespoons fresh lime juice

Instructions:

1. Preheat a grill to medium-high heat.

2. Brush salmon fillets with olive oil and sprinkle with salt and pepper.

3. Grill salmon until cooked through, about five minutes per side.

4. In a medium bowl, combine mango, red onion, cilantro, and lime juice.

5. Serve salmon with mango salsa.

Pre-time: Ten minutes

13. Grilled Vegetable and Hummus Wrap:

Ingredients:

Two whole wheat tortillas

Two tablespoons olive oil

Half cup sliced mushrooms

Half cup diced bell peppers

One-fourth cup diced onion

One-fourth teaspoon salt

One-fourth teaspoon black pepper

One-fourth cup hummus

Instructions:

1. Preheat a grill to medium-high heat.

2. Brush vegetables with olive oil and sprinkle with salt and pepper.

3. Grill vegetables until tender, about five minutes per side.

4. Spread each tortilla with two tablespoons of hummus.

5. Top each with grilled vegetables.

6. Roll up and serve.

Pre-time: Ten minutes

14. Baked Eggplant Parmesan:

Ingredients:

One large eggplant, sliced into half-inch thick rounds

Two tablespoons olive oil

One-fourth teaspoon salt

One-fourth teaspoon black pepper

Half cup marinara sauce

Half cup shredded mozzarella cheese

Instructions:

1. Preheat oven to 375 degrees F.

2. Place eggplant rounds in a single layer on a baking sheet.

3. Apply olive oil to the surface and season with salt and pepper.

4. Bake in preheated oven until eggplant is tender, about fifteen minutes.

5. Spread marinara sauce over eggplant rounds and top with cheese.

6. Bake in preheated oven until cheese is melted and bubbly, about ten minutes more.

Pre-time: Ten minutes

15. Baked Cod with Tomatoes and Capers:

Ingredients:

Two (four-ounce) cod fillets

Two tablespoons olive oil

Two cloves garlic, minced

Two tablespoons fresh lemon juice

Two tablespoons capers

Two tablespoons fresh parsley, chopped

Two tomatoes, diced

One-fourth teaspoon salt

One-fourth teaspoon black pepper

Instructions:

1. Preheat oven to 425 degrees F.

2. Cod fillets should be placed on a baking dish.

3. Drizzle olive oil over the fish.

4. Sprinkle garlic, lemon juice, capers, parsley, tomatoes, salt, and pepper over the fish.

5. Bake in preheated oven until fish flakes easily with a fork, about fifteen minutes.

Pre-time: Ten minutes

16. Roasted Cauliflower and Chickpeas:

Ingredients:

One head cauliflower, cut into florets

Two tablespoons olive oil

Half teaspoon salt

Half teaspoon black pepper

Chickpeas from one (15-ounce) can, drained and rinsed

Instructions:

1. Preheat oven to 400 degrees F.

2. Place cauliflower and chickpeas in a single layer on a baking sheet.

3. Drizzle with olive oil and sprinkle with salt and pepper.

4. Roast in preheated oven until cauliflower is tender and lightly browned, about twenty minutes.

Pre-time: Ten minutes

17. Baked Zucchini Rounds:

Ingredients:

Two zucchinis, sliced into one fourth-inch thick rounds

Two tablespoons olive oil

One-fourth teaspoon salt

One-fourth teaspoon black pepper

Half cup shredded mozzarella cheese

Instructions:

1. Preheat oven to 350 degrees F.

2. Arrange zucchini rounds on a baking sheet.

3. Apply olive oil to the surface and season with salt and pepper.

4. Bake in preheated oven until lightly browned, about ten minutes.

5. Top each round with cheese.

6. Bake in preheated oven until cheese is melted and bubbly, about five minutes more.

Pre-time: Ten minutes

18. Grilled Chicken with Avocado Salsa:

Ingredients:

Two tablespoons olive oil

Two boneless, skinless chicken breasts

One-fourth teaspoon salt

One-fourth teaspoon black pepper

One avocado, diced

One-fourth cup diced red onion

Two tablespoons chopped fresh cilantro

Two tablespoons fresh lime juice

Instructions:

1. Preheat a grill to medium-high heat.

2. Brush chicken with olive oil and sprinkle with salt and pepper.

3. Grill chicken until cooked through, about five minutes per side.

4. In a medium bowl, combine avocado, red onion, cilantro, and lime juice.

5. Serve chicken with avocado salsa.

Pre-time: Ten minutes

19. Quinoa and Black Bean Bowl:

Ingredients:

Two tablespoons olive oil

Half cup diced onion

Half cup diced bell pepper

Two cloves garlic, minced

Half teaspoon cumin

One cup uncooked quinoa

Two cups low-sodium vegetable broth

One (fifteen-ounce) can black beans, drained and rinsed

Instructions:

1. In a medium saucepan, heat the oil over medium heat.

2. Add onion, bell pepper, garlic, and cumin.

3. Cook until vegetables are tender, about five minutes.

4. Add quinoa and vegetable broth.

5. Bring to a boil, reduce heat to low, cover, and simmer until quinoa is cooked through, about fifteen minutes.

6. Stir in black beans and cook until heated through, about five minutes more.

Pre-time: Ten minutes

20. Baked Chicken Breast with Vegetables:

Ingredients:

Two tablespoons olive oil

Two boneless, skinless chicken breasts

One-fourth teaspoon salt

One-fourth teaspoon black pepper

Half cup sliced mushrooms

Half cup diced bell peppers

One-fourth cup diced onion

Instructions:

1. Preheat oven to 375 degrees F.

2. Place chicken breasts in a baking dish.

 3. Brush with olive oil and sprinkle with salt and pepper

. 4. Bake in preheated oven until lightly browned, about fifteen minutes.

5. Add mushrooms, bell peppers, and onion to the baking dish.

6. Bake until chicken is cooked through and vegetables are tender, about fifteen minutes more.

Pre-time: Ten minutes

1. Blueberry & Avocado Yogurt Parfait

Ingredients:

One cup plain Greek yogurt

Half avocado

One-fourth cup blueberries

One-fourth cup slivered almonds

Two tablespoons honey

Instructions:

1. In a bowl, mash the avocado until it is a creamy consistency.

2. Add the yogurt and honey and stir until fully combined.

3. Layer the yogurt mixture, blueberries, and almonds in a parfait glass.

Enjoy!

Pre-time: Ten minutes

2. Peanut Butter Banana Oat Smoothie

Ingredients:

One banana

Half cup almond milk

Two tablespoons oats

Two tablespoons peanut butter

One teaspoon honey

Instructions:

1. All components should be blended in a blender until desire smoothness is achieved.

2. Serve chilled and enjoy!

Pre-time: Five minutes

3. Sweet Potato Fries

Ingredients:

1 large sweet potato

2 tablespoons olive oil

Salt and pepper to taste

Instructions:

1. Preheat oven to 400 degrees F.

2. Peel and slice sweet potato into thin strips.

3. Toss sweet potato strips in olive oil, salt and pepper.

4. Place on a parchment-lined baking sheet and bake for 20 minutes.

5. Serve hot and enjoy!

Pre-time: Ten minutes

4. Baked Apple Chips

Ingredients:

Two large apples

Two teaspoons cinnamon

Two tablespoons honey

Instructions:

1. Preheat oven to 375 degrees F.

2. Core and slice apples into thin slices.

3. Mix together cinnamon and honey in a bowl.

4. Dip apple slices in the cinnamon and honey mixture and place on a parchment-lined baking sheet.

5. Until golden brown is reached, bake for twenty minutes..

 Enjoy!

Pre-time: Fifteen minutes

5. Greek Yogurt Fruit Dip

Ingredients:

One cup plain Greek yogurt

 Two tablespoons honey

Two tablespoons lemon juice

 Half teaspoon vanilla extract

Instructions:

1. Mix all ingredients in a bowl until everything is well blended.

2. Serve with fresh fruit of your choice and enjoy!

Pre-time: Five minutes

6. Banana Oat Muffins

Ingredients:

One cup oats

One banana

One egg

Two tablespoons honey

Two tablespoons almond milk

One teaspoon baking powder

Instructions:

1. Preheat oven to 350 degrees F.

2. Mash banana in a bowl and mix in the other ingredients until fully combined.

3. Cooking spray should be used to grease a muffin pan.

4. Fill the muffin tins with the batter and bake for fifteen minutes.

5. Serve warm and enjoy!

Pre-time: Ten minutes

7. Avocado Egg Toast

Ingredients:

One slice whole wheat toast, half avocado and one egg

Instructions:

1. Toast the slice of whole wheat toast.

2. Meanwhile, mash avocado in a bowl.

3. Fry the egg in a skillet.

4. Spread the mashed avocado on the toast and top with the fried egg.

5. Enjoy!

Pre-time: Ten minutes

8. Baked Sweet Potato Fries

Ingredients:

2 large sweet potatoes

2 tablespoons olive oil

Salt and pepper to taste

Instructions:

1. Preheat oven to 400 degrees F.

2. Peel and slice sweet potatoes into thin strips.

3. Toss sweet potato strips in olive oil, salt, and pepper.

4. Place on a parchment-lined baking sheet and bake for twenty minutes.

5. Serve hot and enjoy!

Pre-time: Ten minutes

9. Cottage Cheese & Fruit Bowl

Ingredients:

One cup cottage cheese, half cup fresh fruit of your choice

Instructions:

1. In a bowl, mix together cottage cheese and fruit.

2. Enjoy!

Pre-time: Five minutes

10. Trail Mix

Ingredients:

One cup almonds

Half cup dried cranberries

Half cup dark chocolate chips

Half cup pumpkin seeds

Instructions:

1. Mix all ingredients in a bowl until everything is well blended.

2. Serve and enjoy!

Pre-time: Five minutes

11. Overnight Oats

Ingredients:

One cup oats

One cup almond milk

Two tablespoons honey

One teaspoon cinnamon

Instructions:

1. Mix all ingredients in a bowl until everything is well blended.

2. Refrigerate overnight.

3. Serve chilled and enjoy!

Pre-time: Five minutes

12. Roasted Chickpeas

Ingredients:

One can chickpeas

Two tablespoons olive oil

Salt and pepper to taste

Instructions:

1. Preheat oven to 375 degrees F.

2. Rinse and drain chickpeas.

3. Place chickpeas on a parchment-lined baking sheet and toss in olive oil, salt, and pepper.

4. Bake for twenty five minutes or until golden brown.

5. Serve hot and enjoy!

Pre-time: Five minutes

13. Frozen Yogurt Bites

Ingredients:

One cup plain Greek yogurt

Half cup fresh fruit of your choice

Two tablespoons honey

Instructions:

1. Use parchment paper to line a baking sheet.

2. In a bowl, mix together yogurt, fruit, and honey until fully combined.

3. Drop spoonfuls of the mixture onto the baking sheet and freeze for one hour.

4. Serve frozen and enjoy!

Pre-time: Fifteen minutes

14. Sweet Potato Toast

Ingredients:

One large sweet potato

Two tablespoons olive oil

Salt and pepper to taste

Instructions:

1. Preheat oven to 400 degrees F.

2. Slice sweet potato into thin slices.

3. Toss sweet potato slices in olive oil, salt, and pepper.

4. Place on a parchment-lined baking sheet and bake for twenty minutes.

5. Serve hot and enjoy!

Pre-time: Ten minutes

15. Veggie Pita Pockets

Ingredients:

Two whole wheat pitas

Half cup shredded cheese

One-fourth cup sliced bell peppers

One-fourth cup sliced cucumbers

Instructions:

1. Preheat oven to 375 degrees F.

2. Cut each pita into half and fill with shredded cheese, bell peppers, and cucumbers.

3. Place on a parchment-lined baking sheet and bake for 10 minutes.

4. Serve warm and enjoy!

Pre-time: Ten minutes

16. Grilled Cheese Sandwich

Ingredients:

Two slices whole wheat bread

Two tablespoons butter

Two slices cheese

Instructions:

1. Heat a skillet over medium heat.

2. Spread butter on one side of each slice of bread.

3. Place one slice of bread, butter side down, in the skillet and top with cheese.

4. Top with the remaining slice of bread, butter side up.

5. Grill for two-three minutes per side or until golden brown.

6. Serve warm and enjoy!

Pre-time: Five minutes

17. Hummus & Veggies

Ingredients:

One cup hummus

 One cup sliced vegetables of your choice

Instructions:

1. In a bowl, mix together hummus and vegetables.

2. Enjoy!

Pre-time: Five minutes

18. Fruit & Cheese Plate

Ingredients:

One cup fresh fruit of your choice

 One cup cheese of your choice

Instructions:

1. Arrange the fruit and cheese on a plate.

2. Serve and enjoy!

Pre-time: Five minutes

19. Popcorn

Ingredients:

3 tablespoons popcorn kernels

2 tablespoons olive oil

Salt and pepper to taste

Instructions:

1. Add olive oil to a big pot that's already at medium heat.

2. Add popcorn kernels and cover with lid.

3. Shake pot back and forth over the burner until kernels start to pop.

4. Once popping slows down, remove from heat and season with salt and pepper.

5. Serve and enjoy!

Pre-time: Five minutes

20. Frozen Grapes

Ingredients:

One cup grapes

Instructions:

1. Place grapes on a parchment-lined baking sheet and freeze for One hour.

2. Serve frozen and enjoy!

Pre-time: Five minutes

1. Banana Split Oatmeal Bowl:

Ingredients:

Half cup rolled oats

Half cup almond milk

Half teaspoon vanilla extract

Half banana, sliced

One-fourth cup low-fat vanilla Greek yogurt

One tablespoon honey

One-fourth cup fresh strawberries, sliced

One-fourth cup fresh blueberries

One tablespoon chopped walnuts

Instructions:

1. In a medium-sized saucepan, combine oats, almond milk, and vanilla extract. Bring to a boil over medium-high heat. Reduce heat to low and simmer, stirring occasionally, until oats are cooked through, about five minutes.

2. Divide cooked oatmeal among two bowls.

3. Top each bowl with banana slices, yogurt, honey, strawberries, blueberries, and walnuts. Serve warm.

Pre-time: Ten minutes

2. Avocado and Almond Butter Toast:

Ingredients:

Two slices whole wheat bread

Two tablespoons almond butter

Half avocado, sliced

One-fourth teaspoon ground cinnamon

One tablespoon honey

Instructions:

1. Toast bread until lightly golden brown.

2. Spread each toast with one tablespoon almond butter.

3. Top with avocado slices, cinnamon, and honey.

Pre-time: Five minutes

3. Apple Pie Yogurt Bowl:

Ingredients:

Half cup plain Greek yogurt

One-fourth cup unsweetened applesauce

One-fourth teaspoon ground cinnamon

One-fourth teaspoon ground nutmeg

Half apple, diced

One tablespoon chopped walnuts

One tablespoon raisins

Instructions:

1. In a medium bowl, combine yogurt, applesauce, cinnamon, and nutmeg. Stir until well combined.

2. Divide yogurt mixture among two bowls.

3. Top each bowl with diced apples, walnuts, and raisins. Serve chilled.

Pre-time: Ten minutes

4. Peanut Butter and Banana Smoothie Bowl:

Ingredients:

Half banana

Half cup almond milk

One tablespoon peanut butter

One-fourth teaspoon ground cinnamon

One-fourth teaspoon ground nutmeg

One-fourth cup granola

Instructions:

1. Place banana, almond milk, peanut butter, cinnamon, and nutmeg in a blender. Blend until smooth.

2. Divide smoothie among two bowls.

3. Top each bowl with granola. Serve chilled.

Pre-time: Five minutes

5. Baked Apple Chips:

Ingredients:

Two apples, cored and sliced thin

One tablespoon honey

One-fourth teaspoon ground cinnamon

Instructions:

1. Preheat oven to 250°F.

2. Use parchment paper to line a baking sheet.

3. Arrange apple slices on prepared baking sheet.

4. Drizzle honey and sprinkle cinnamon over apples.

5. Bake for one hour, flipping halfway through, until apples are lightly browned and crisp.

6. Let cool before serving.

Pre-time: Fifteen minutes

6. Frozen Banana Bites:

Ingredients:

Three bananas, sliced

One-fourth cup melted dark chocolate chips

One tablespoon chopped walnuts

Instructions:

1. Use parchment paper to line a baking sheet.

2. Arrange banana slices on prepared baking sheet.

3. Drizzle melted chocolate over bananas. Sprinkle with walnuts.

4. Freeze for one hour until firm.

5. Store in an airtight container in the freezer.

Pre-time: Fifteen minutes

7. Chocolate Overnight Oats:

Ingredients:

Half cup rolled oats

Half cup almond milk

Half teaspoon vanilla extract

One tablespoon cocoa powder

One tablespoon honey

One-fourth cup fresh strawberries, diced

Instructions:

1. In a medium bowl, combine oats, almond milk, and vanilla extract. Stir until well combined.

2. Stir in cocoa powder and honey.

3. Divide oatmeal among two jars or containers.

4. Top each jar with strawberries.

5. Refrigerate overnight. Serve chilled.

Pre-time: Five minutes

8. Peanut Butter and Banana Wrap:

Ingredients:

Two whole wheat tortillas

Two tablespoons peanut butter

Half banana, sliced

One-fourth teaspoon ground cinnamon

Instructions:

1. Spread each tortilla with one tablespoon peanut butter.

2. Top each tortilla with banana slices and cinnamon.

3. Roll up each tortilla and cut in half.

4. Serve chilled or at room temperature.

Pre-time: Five minutes

9. Chocolate Dipped Strawberries:

Ingredients:

Half cup dark chocolate chips

One-fourth cup coconut oil

One pint fresh strawberries

Instructions:

1. Use parchment paper to line a baking sheet.

2. Put chocolate chips and coconut oil in a bowl that can go in the microwave. Heat in fifteen-second intervals, stirring after each interval, until melted and smooth.

3. Dip each strawberry in melted chocolate, swirling to coat completely.

4. Place dipped strawberries on prepared baking sheet.

5. Refrigerate for one hour until chocolate is set.

Pre-time: Fifteen minutes

10. Coconut Yogurt Parfait:

Ingredients:

Half cup plain Greek yogurt

One-fourth cup shredded coconut

One-fourth cup fresh blueberries

One tablespoon honey

Instructions:

1. In a medium bowl, combine yogurt and coconut. Stir until well combined.

2. Divide yogurt mixture among two cups or jars.

3. Top each cup with blueberries and honey. Serve chilled.

Pre-time: Five minutes

1. Pineapple Coconut Smoothie:

Ingredients:

One cup fresh pineapple chunks

Half cup coconut water

One-fourth cup light coconut milk

One scoop vanilla protein powder

Half teaspoon ground cinnamon

Instructions:

1. To make everything completely smooth, put everything in a blender and blend for smoothness.

2. Pour into a tall glass and enjoy!

Pre-Time: Five minutes

2. Peanut Butter Banana Smoothie:

Ingredients:

One frozen banana

Half cup almond milk

One tablespoon peanut butter

One scoop vanilla protein powder

Half teaspoon ground cinnamon

Instructions:

1. In a blender, combine all ingredients and blend until perfectly smoothness is reached.

2. Pour into a tall glass and enjoy!

Pre-Time: Five minutes

3. Strawberry Oat Smoothie:

Ingredients:

One cup frozen strawberries

Half cup almond milk

One-fourth cup oats

One scoop vanilla protein powder

Half teaspoon ground cinnamon

Instructions:

1. All components should be processed in a blender until they are perfectly smooth.

2. Pour into a tall glass and enjoy!

Pre-Time: Five minutes

4. Raspberry Mango Smoothie:

Ingredients:

One cup frozen raspberries

Half cup coconut milk

One-fourth cup mango chunks

One scoop vanilla protein powder

Half teaspoon ground cinnamon

Instructions:

1 In a blender, combine all ingredients and process until perfectly smooth.

2. Pour into a tall glass and enjoy!

Pre-Time: Five minutes

5. Blueberry Acai Smoothie:

Ingredients:

One cup frozen blueberries

Half cup almond milk

One-fourth cup acai berry puree

One scoop vanilla protein powder

Half teaspoon ground cinnamon

Instructions:

1. All ingredients should be mashed in a blender until they are perfectly smooth.

2. Pour into a tall glass and enjoy!

Pre-Time: Five minutes

6. Green Apple Smoothie:

Ingredients:

One green apple, cored and sliced

Half cup almond milk

One-fourth cup spinach

One scoop vanilla protein powder

Half teaspoon ground cinnamon

Instructions:

1. All ingredients should be blended in a blender until smooth.

2. Pour into a tall glass and enjoy!

Pre-Time: Five minutes

7. Kale Avocado Smoothie:

Ingredients:

One cup kale

Half cup almond milk

One-fourth avocado

One scoop vanilla protein powder

Half teaspoon ground cinnamon

Instructions:

1. All ingredients should be thoroughly smooth after being processed in a blender.

2. Pour into a tall glass and enjoy!

Pre-Time: Five minutes

8. Carrot Orange Smoothie:

Ingredients:

Half cup fresh carrot juice

Half cup orange juice

One-fourth cup Greek yogurt

One scoop vanilla protein powder

Half teaspoon ground cinnamon

Instructions:

1 To make everything completely smooth, put everything in a blender and blend for smoothness.

2. Pour into a tall glass and enjoy!

Pre-Time: Five minutes

9. Chocolate Banana Smoothie:

Ingredients:

One frozen banana

Half cup almond milk

One-fourth cup cocoa powder

One scoop vanilla protein powder

Half teaspoon ground cinnamon

Instructions:

1. To make everything completely smooth, put everything in a blender and blend.

2. Pour into a tall glass and enjoy!

Pre-Time: Five minutes

10. Beet Almond Smoothie:

Ingredients:

Half cup beet juice

Half cup almond milk

One-fourth cup almonds

One scoop vanilla protein powder

Half teaspoon ground cinnamon

Instructions:

1. All ingredients should be processed in a blender until smoothness is reached.

2. Pour into a tall glass and enjoy!

Pre-Time: Five minutes

11. Banana Coconut Smoothie:

Ingredients:

One frozen banana

Half cup coconut milk

One-fourth cup shredded coconut

One scoop vanilla protein powder

Half teaspoon ground cinnamon

Instructions:

1. Blend all ingredients in a blender until desire smoothness is reached.

2. Pour into a tall glass and enjoy!

Pre-Time: Five minutes

12. Pear Ginger Smoothie:

Ingredients:

One pear, cored and sliced

Half cup almond milk

One-fourth teaspoon fresh grated ginger

One scoop vanilla protein powder

Half teaspoon ground cinnamon

Instructions:

1. All ingredients should be processed in a blender until desire smoothness is met

2. Pour into a tall glass and enjoy!

Pre-Time: Five minutes

13. Kiwi Mango Smoothie:

Ingredients:

One kiwi, peeled and sliced

Half cup coconut milk

One-fourth cup mango chunks

One scoop vanilla protein powder

Half teaspoon ground cinnamon

Instructions:

1. All ingredients should be thoroughly blended in a blender until desire smooth.

2. Pour into a tall glass and enjoy!

Pre-Time: Five minutes

14. Cucumber Apple Smoothie:

Ingredients:

Half cucumber, peeled and diced

Half cup apple juice

One-fourth cup Greek yogurt

One scoop vanilla protein powder

Half teaspoon ground cinnamon

Instructions:

1. In a blender, combine all ingredients and process until perfectly creamy.

2. Pour into a tall glass and enjoy!

Pre-Time: Five minutes

CONCLUSION

Eating yourself thin is not an easy task, nor is it a quick one. It requires dedication, consistency, and a willingness to make changes to your lifestyle and diet. However, it is possible to achieve a healthy, fit body by eating the right foods and exercising regularly. With the right tools and knowledge, you can make the changes necessary to achieve your desired healthy weight. Eating yourself thin is a process that can take time, but the health and fitness benefits are worth the effort.

www.ingramcontent.com/pod-product-compliance
Lightning Source LLC
Chambersburg PA
CBHW061616250726
48653CB00016B/1971